W9-AVC-490

THE FANTASY BOOK

A JOURNEY

*W*ith this book begins a **journey**

when you come upon a fantasy

that you wish to **explore**

place the bookmark

close the cover

and **leave** it for me

as a silent **invitation** . . .

Research by Norma Wilson
Design consulting and quote sourcing by Susan Ellinger
Image and production consulting by Linda Marso
Rights and clearances by Nancy Galdo and Silvia Royer

PHOTOGRAPHY

Photographer: Michele Clement
Photo agent: Norman Maslov
Assistant photographers: Michael Bennett
and Toni Scott
Photo assistants: Anthony Gamboa and
Sapasorn Ridhikerd
Archivist and retoucher: Norberto Melendez
Wardrobe and prop stylist: Lisa Fremont
Assistant stylist: Lena Young
Linens by Erica Tanov (Berkeley, CA)
Hair and makeup: Manjari from Koko
Represents, Ivan Mendoza, and Matt
Monzon
Photo shoot production: Aneata Hagy and
Fiona O'Connor
Interns: Maya Linke, Nancy Wolf, Heather
Knappe, and Pat Mazzera
Talent: Alice-Gray Lewis, Brian Toolajian,
and Seamus Lynch
Illustrated postcards in Part IV photograph:
Scott Miller

ILLUSTRATIONS

"Write Me a Love Letter" collage by
Gerry Safulko
"One Romantic Evening" collage by Rinat
Aldema, David Russell, and Gary Silver;
original line drawing courtesy of Nik
Douglas and Penny Slinger
"Surprise Me" collage by Gerry Safulko
"Positions" collage by Rinat Aldema, David
Russell, and Gary Silver; original line
drawings courtesy of Nik Douglas and
Penny Slinger
"One Then Nine" illustration courtesy of
Nik Douglas and Penny Slinger
"Spanking" artwork by Grace Moon

Every attempt has been made to credit the
proper sources for all quotations and artwork. If you feel that someone has been
overlooked, please contact the publisher
regarding future editions.

www.TheFantasyBook.com

Copyright © 2006 by Noise Production,
Inc. and LP Communications, Inc.
Photographs copyright © 2006 by
Michele Clement

All rights reserved.

Published in the United States by Clarkson
Potter/Publishers, an imprint of the Crown
Publishing Group, a division of Random
House, Inc., New York.
www.crownpublishing.com
www.clarksonpotter.com

Clarkson N. Potter is a trademark and Potter
and colophon are registered trademarks of
Random House, Inc.

Library of Congress Cataloging-in-
Publication Data is available upon request.

ISBN-13: 978-0-307-23606-7

Printed in Singapore

10 9 8 7 6 5 4 3 2 1

First Edition

THE FANTASY BOOK

GARY SILVER
DAVID RUSSELL

PHOTOGRAPHS BY MICHELE CLEMENT

CLARKSON POTTER/PUBLISHERS
NEW YORK

INSTRUCTIONS

THE BOOKMARK

Use the bookmark to secretly share fantasies with your partner. Place it at
the fantasy you would like to fulfill, close the cover, and leave the book where
your partner will discover it. When your partner finds the book with your
fantasy selected, he or she will know your desire.

THE ENVELOPES

If you place the bookmark at one of the fantasies that contains an envelope, write
down your specific request and leave it in the envelope for your partner to find.

AN IMPORTANT NOTE

When engaging in fantasy play, it is important to put the safety and
well-being of your partner first and never do anything that would endanger
either of you. Due to the very nature of fantasy play, the authors and the
publisher cannot accept liability for any loss or risk incurred by the use or
application of the contents of this book.

CONTENTS

PART I SEDUCE ME

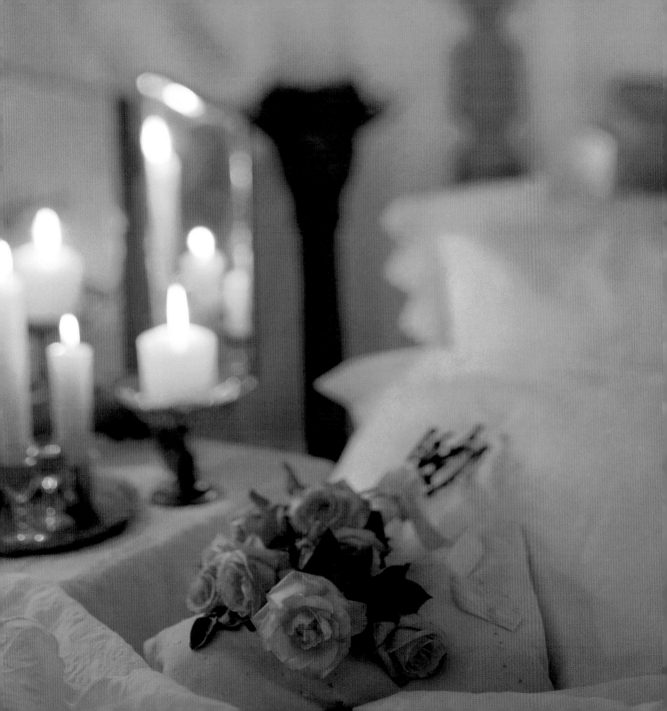

A young bachelor of an adventurous nature comes home at
dawn, having spent the night in some amorous encounter . . .
He immediately draws his inkstone to him and, after carefully
rubbing it with ink, starts to write his next-morning letter. He
does not let his brush run down the paper in a careless scrawl,
but puts himself heart and soul into the calligraphy . . .

Then he makes arrangements for delivering his letter. . . . he
takes the trouble to get up and select a pageboy who seems
suitable for the task. . . . the messenger returns . . . and nods
encouragingly to his master, who thereupon instantly interrupts
his recitation and, with what might strike one as sinful haste,
transfers his attention to the lady's reply.

Sei Shonagon
The Pillow Book of Sei Shonagon
(Japan, tenth century)

*I*f I were to find **an envelope**

with my name **written in your hand**

I would savor the weight and touch of it

and wonder what **persuasive words** lay

inside

Pleasure has endowed the dance with a powerful
charm. The hands which
touch each other, the arms
which entwine, operate like conductors of
electricity . . .

And how can one's sensibility
not be affected by the
delicious sensations which we feel? . . .

The ears are profoundly
touched by the sounds of the
instruments . . . the sense of
smell is conquered by the
variety of perfumes—and
when all these delights are
seconded by the pleasures
of the dance itself, their
combination is virtually irresistible . . .

Only if one has never danced
with the object of one's affection
can one ignore the force of this
all too powerful magnetism.

M. L. E. Moreau de Saint-Méry
Report on the colonies to the people of Europe, 1796

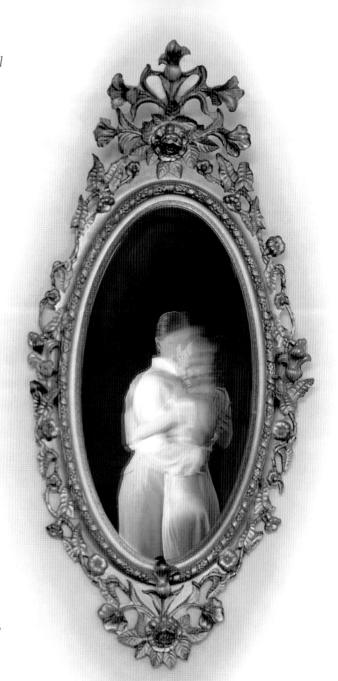

I'd like to feel your warm

body pressed against me

swaying to the music

of **our rhythm**

turning to the rhythm

of **our universe**

One day we read,
for pastime and
sweet cheer,

Of Lancelot,
how he found
Love tyrannous:

We were alone,
and without
any fear.

Our eyes were
drawn together,
reading thus,

Full oft, and
still our cheeks
would pale and glow;

But one sole
point it was that
conquered us.

For when we
read of that
great lover, how

He kissed the
smile which he
had longed to win,

Then he whom
naught can sever
from me now

For ever,
kissed my mouth,
all quivering.

A pandar was
the book,
and he that writ.

Upon that day
we read no
more therein.

Dante Alighieri
Inferno, Canto V

I close my eyes
        and listen to the
        sound of your voice

entering my mind
engaging my body
breaking through

my inhibitions
        with the power of words

                read to me

a story about anything
perhaps about us

Splendid Divalgiri, or wall lights, should gleam around the hall, reflected by a hundred mirrors, whilst both man and woman should contend against any reserve, or false shame, giving themselves up in complete nakedness to unrestrained voluptuousness, upon a high and handsome bedstead, raised on tall legs, furnished with many pillows, and covered by a rich chatra, or canopy; the sheets being besprinkled with flowers and the coverlet scented by burning luscious incense, such as aloes and other fragrant woods. In such a place, let the man, ascending the throne of love, enjoy the woman in ease and comfort, gratifying his and her every wish and every whim.

Ananga Ranga

(India, twelfth century)

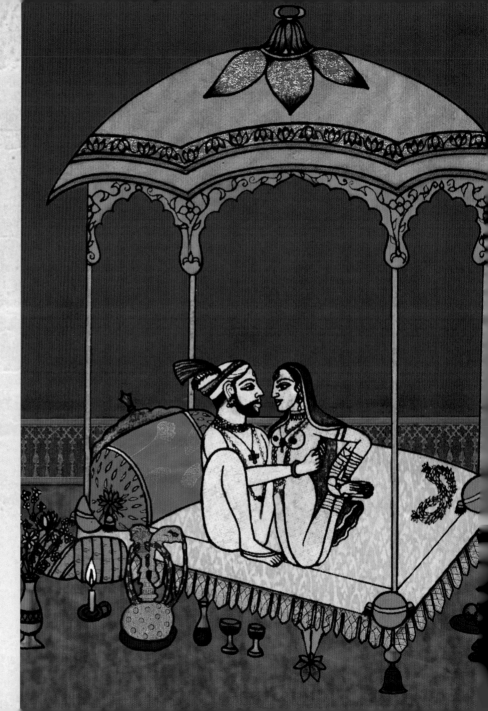

*S*urrender **an evening**

           an evening without time

an evening without end

           Prepare for this **special night**

           and let us take our fill **until morning**

If I had my way we'd sleep every night all wrapped around each other like hibernating rattlesnakes.

William S. Burroughs

*I*n the stillness, under the same cover—we lie nested,

safe in the balance where dreams meet sleep.

so intimate that your hand upon my chest is my hand,
so intimate that when I fall asleep it is your eyes that close.

Pablo Neruda
"Sonnet XVII"

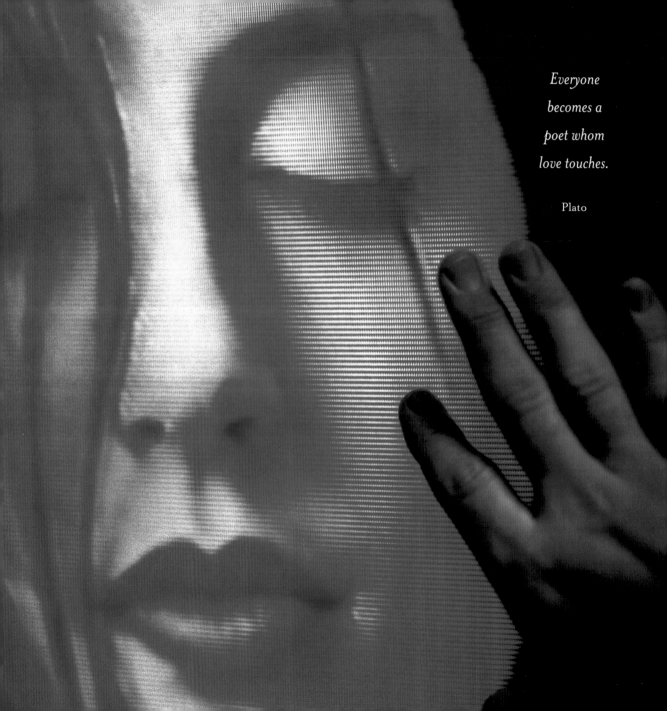

Everyone

becomes a

poet whom

love touches.

Plato

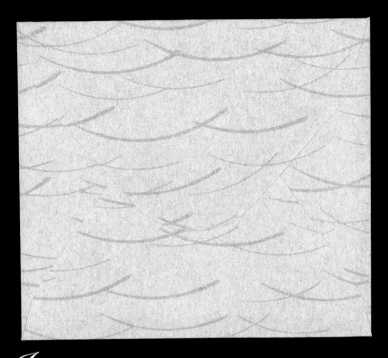

*I*n the Japanese pillow books of the Kamakura period,

there is often mention of a **poetic exchange** between lovers.

They would send each other half-completed poems, inviting

their partner to provide the missing verse. In the envelope,

I have left you the first three lines of a haiku.

E-mail me your response.

Woman is like a fruit which

Will not yield its sweetness until

You rub it between your hands

Sheik Nefzawi
The Perfumed Garden

My **secrets**

are hidden in the most unexpected places,

silent, waiting to be unlocked.

Your hands

hold the key,

the unspoken poetry of heat and motion.

He brought volcanic pumice
stone for my feet, his mother's
homemade tropical shampoo
for my hair, and coconut
massage oil for my sunburned
skin. Because he was deeply
interested in geology, he made a
life-size topographical map of my
body, naming his favorite places—
my back, hands, and neck—after
mountains and velleys he'd
studied on maps of the ancient
world. I wrote him primitive
poetry, reciting it in our bath as
we faced each other encircled by
candles. In our glowing water
cave, we were two initiates,
learning the luxurious language
of **touch** and **time.**

Brenda Peterson

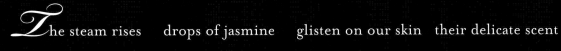

The steam rises   drops of jasmine   glisten on our skin   their delicate scent

arousing our senses

The air is deep   rose petals   float on the surface   reflecting their timeless

message of desire

23

No one in the world
could respond more
keenly to the
deepest and most
secret gropings of
my soul.

No musical
dedication
has ever been
more seriously meant.

It was spoken not
only on my part
but on yours;
the symphony was
not, in truth, mine
but ours.

Pyotr Tchaikovsky to Countess Nadezhda von Meck

I find myself

        thinking of you

     imagining you are

        thinking about me

Surprise me . . .

     perhaps with flowers and chocolates, a love poem,
     or something hypnotic and seductive
     like a **musical compilation**
        for us to make love to

Then you rose into my life
Like a promised sunrise
Brightening my days with the light in your eyes . . .

Maya Angelou
"Where We Belong, A Duet"

I awaken unexpectedly at **dawn**

your breath no longer soft against my skin

how quietly you slipped from beneath the covers

to prepare this **celebration**

of our waking **together**

PART II AROUSE ME

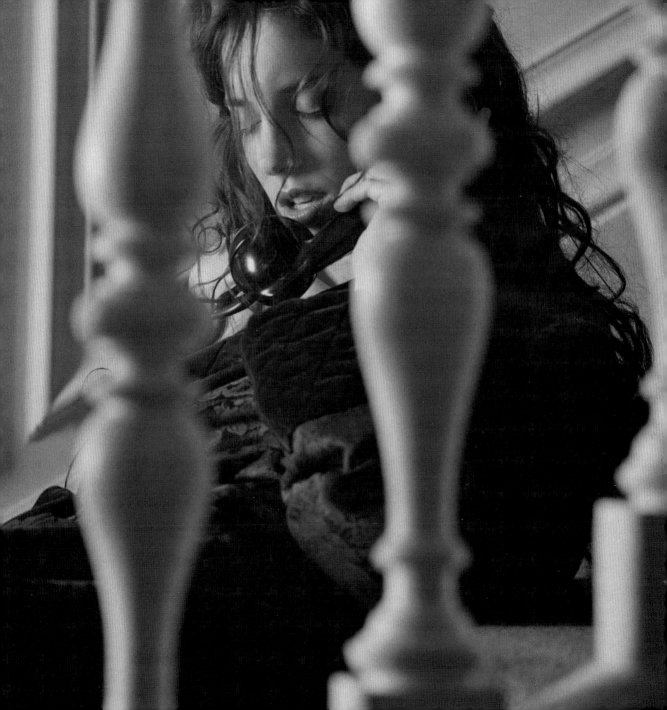

He took off my dress, slowly. Then he stretched me out on
the warm tiles and, with the shower still running,
began planting kisses all over my body.

Alina Reyes

I want to feel your lips

teasing

    tasting

        exploring

    like an endless stream flowing

down

    my

        body

She was not quite naked

but this was much worse. She was

far more indecent,

much more shockingly

indecent this way than

if she had been

simply naked.

Jules Barbey d'Aurevilly
Feu d'Amour

*I*magine yourself through my eyes when **I envision you** in . . .

Massage her body
with sweet sandal-oil.

Soon she won't object
to fingers that stray
under her skirt-hem
and linger at her
lightly knotted
waistband;

When her eyes
are dreamy and
her breathing's harsh,
send the servants away.

*The Love Teachings
of Kama Sutra*

Translated by
Indra Sinha

*E*verywhere our bodies **naked** and entwined

    glistening

        dripping

        reflecting

exploring every curve and contour as we slide

        first up then down

    gleaming

        glorified

        shimmering from the **heat**

Am I going too slow for you?

       No no, keep going, that's fine.

*Oh, I love moving my hands over
you under your loose shirt, I love
that. I'd slide my hands around over
your stomach, so that my fingertips
met, and feel it pull in, and slide up
slowly along your ribs, and when I got
to where the curves of your breasts
started, I would trace them around,
out to the sides, back to the middle,
and I would pass just my fingertips
up between your breasts, up along your
breastbone, pushing under the loose
bra, and then one finger even higher, along
your voice box, to where your chin starts,
and you'd lean your head back and I
would be able to smell your hair, and
then I'd pull back down, deliberately
avoiding your breasts.*

      *And I would stand up, she said, and turn
around so I'm facing you, with my shins
touching the armchair, and I'd undo
the button of my pants.*

Nicholson Baker
Vox

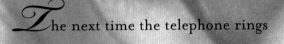

The next time the telephone rings

maybe it will be you

behind **mysterious whispers**

beyond the power of **touch**

I await your call

When you've reached the place, where a girl loves to be touched, don't let

modesty prevent you touching her.

Ovid

Ars Amatoria II

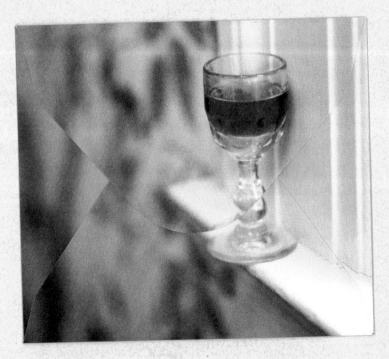

*I*n the envelope I have left you a love potion

    a list of places where **I would love to be touched**
    and particular ways that I would like you to touch them.

    Mix them **seductively** to increase the power of your spell.

*Time is dilated, pleasure is extended, all
the senses are opened to this experience,
and suddenly the bodies truly take their
place in space. Play, laughter, breathing,
the shuddering of limbs, all tend toward
opening. The eyes, the intimate organs, the
heart all come alive. The whole chemistry
of the body is altered, the mind eases, and
the brain teems. The skin softens and
exhales its perfume. At this moment only,
two bodies communicate deeply and there
is something of the divine in the
sexual relationship.*

Daniel Odier
Tantric Quest

THE LOVERS' DANCE

*C*enturies ago in Brazil,
    couples would learn how to touch
    each other in an erotic ritual known as
    á dança dos amantes.

One of the lovers
    would stand behind the other,
    and begin **slowly caressing** them.
    The partner would then take
    the other's hands and gently guide
    the touch, **silently teaching**
    where **pleasures** lay,
    until the dance became
    an exultation of
    learning and **desire.**

Stand behind me,
    and give me your hands . . .

JEANNE: *I don't know what to call you.*

PAUL: *I don't have a name.*

JEANNE: *You want to know mine?*

PAUL: *No! No, I don't—I don't want to know your name. You don't have a name, and I don't have a name either. No names here. Not one name.*

Bernardo Bertolucci
Last Tango in Paris

EROTIC MOVIE

FAIS L'AMOUR AVEC

make love to

MOI AVEC TA JUPE REMONTÉE

me with your skirt hiked up

ET BAS DESCENDUS

and stockings down

ENTRE MES CUISSES OUVERTES

between my open thighs

LAISSANT TA LANGUE

allowing your tongue

DOUCEMENT

softly

COMME UNE PLUME
CONTRE MA DURE

*like a feather
against my hard*

TOUCHE SATISFAIT TON
BESOIN DE NE SENTIR

*touch satisfies
your need to feel*

RIEN ENTRE NOUS DEUX.

nothing between us.

*I*magine a movie **so passionate** that
you find yourself thinking about us

let's watch an erotic movie

My cloak has only to fall in order that thou mayest discover a succession of mysteries.

Gustave Flaubert

*U*nderstand that you are **my fantasy**
and I live for the moment of your slow revelation

let the power of **your movements**
overwhelm my defenses

as you slowly unveil
the mysteries of **your body**

Recipe

INGREDIENTS

Forty 10-ounce bags of marshmallows
One 24-ounce squeeze bottle of chocolate syrup

DIRECTIONS

1. Fill the bathtub with marshmallows.

2. Warm the chocolate syrup.

3. Escort your partner to the tub and
   help him or her in.

4. Start with chocolate body painting
   and lingering kisses.

5. When you're ready, get in
   and go full-on with the chocolate.

6. Begin feeding each other
   marshmallows.

7. When it's time to rinse off, turn on the
   water and let the tub fill up.

8. Lie back and relax as the
   marshmallows melt around you.

EASY CLEAN-UP

Continue to run the hot water
until the marshmallows have dissolved.

When is food magic? What are the common
denominators? Certainly, when food is the result of
a brilliant and obsessive personal vision, it can take on
mystical, magical aspects.

　　At their best, chefs like to consider themselves alchemists.

Anthony Bourdain
A Cook's Tour

MARSHMALLOW LOVE TUB

*P*icture
a bathtub
full
full
full
of you and me
and
marshmallows
marshmallows
marshmallows
and
chocolate syrup
dripping
down my
sticky
lick it!
body

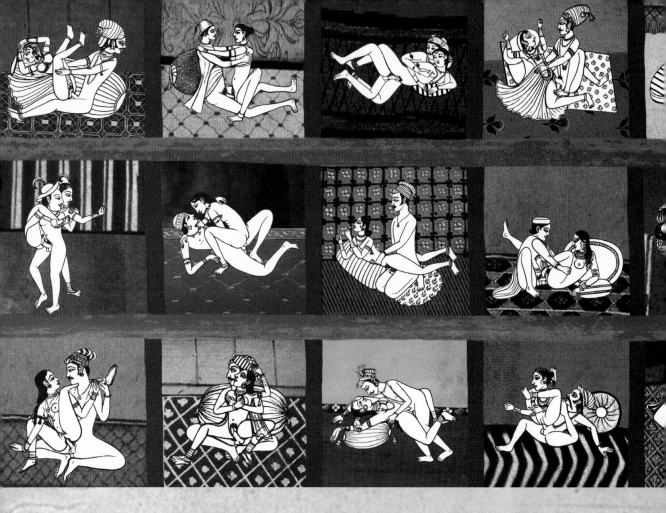

When the red flower shows its beauty
and exhales its heady perfume,
while she stays with you in the night
and you play and take your pleasure with her,
pointing at the pictures you follow their sequence.

Chang Heng Ch'i-pieu
(A.D. 78)

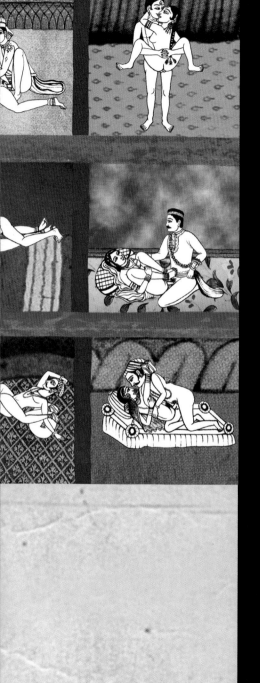

POSITIONS

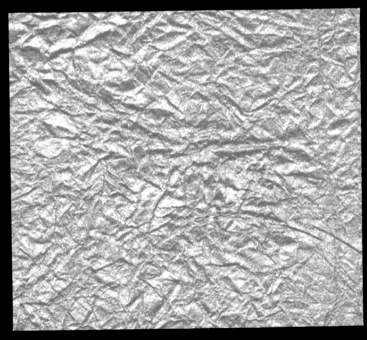

*T*hink of all the **different positions**

we could **explore** . . .

In the envelope, you will find my choices.

PART III THRILL ME

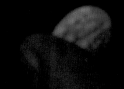

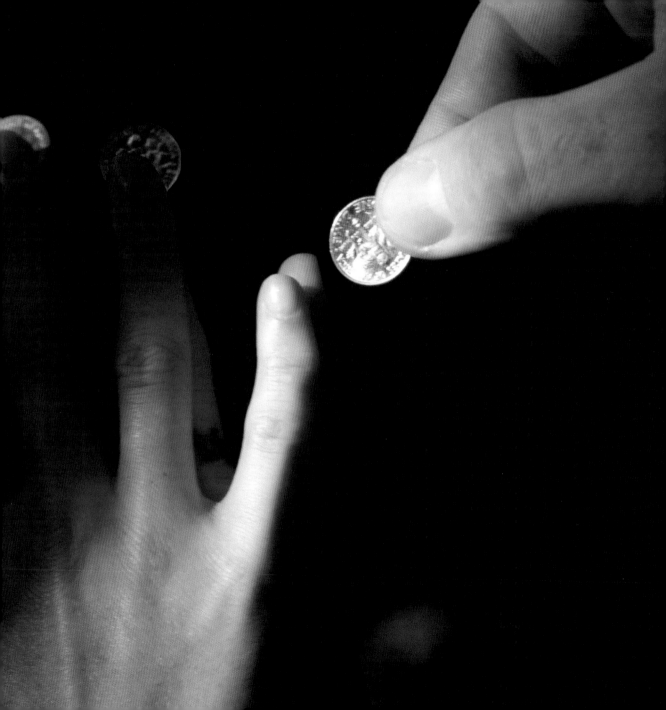

I find her in a noisy crowd.
We look for a secluded spot.

     Fallen blossoms are our
     mattress . . .

     Teased, her face blushes deeply,
Nowhere to hide,
She closes her starry eyes . . .

yen-shih poem
author unknown
(China, twelfth century)

*N*ot far beyond the circle where we **make love** lies a backdrop for our desire . . .

Perhaps . . .

in a hot tub

under the stars

in a hammock

surrounded by wilderness

in a car

on a beach at sunset

or quickly in an elevator

Take me **in another world** . . .

I caress his body amid the sound, the passers-by.

The sea, the immensity,

gathering, receding,

returning.

I asked him to do it again

and again.

Do it to me. And he did.

Marguerite Duras
The Lover

Then came the game of tongues, which I shall not
explain because it is well known to all true lovers.

It so chanced that a fine oyster slipped from its
shell as I was placing it between Emile's lips.

It fell on to her breast, and she would have recovered
it with her fingers; but I claimed the right of regaining
it myself, and she had to unlace her bodice to let me
do so. I got hold of the oyster with my lips, but
did so in such a manner as to prevent her
suspecting that I had taken any extraordinary
pleasure in the act . . . .

"I want my oyster," said I.

"Take it, then."

There was no need to tell me twice.
I unlaced her corset in such
a way as to make it fall still
lower, bewailing the
necessity of having to
search for it with
my hands.

When I had got the
oyster again I could
restrain myself no more,
and affixing my lips to
one of the blossoms of
her breast I sucked it
with a voluptuous
pleasure, which is beyond
all description. She was astonished,
but evidently moved, and I did not leave
her till my enjoyment was complete.

Casanova
*The Complete Memoirs of Jacques
Casanova de Seingalt 1725–1798*

*T*his is your invitation to a very special tasting.

Lovers in the seventeenth century would dine on **aphrodisiacal meals** prepared according to The Doctrine of Signatures, which linked certain foods by their color, shape, and texture to different **sensual responses** in the body.

At the end of the meal, one of the lovers would lie **naked** across the table, surrounded by candles, while the other ate dessert from their body.
If you like, we can skip right to **dessert**.

In fact, though their acquaintance had been so short,

they had guessed, as always happens between lovers,

everything of any importance about each other

in two seconds at the utmost . . .

Virginia Woolf
Orlando

*L*ast night as I slept
        you entered my **dreams**
                and we had an **illicit affair.**

First we were a French aristocrat and his courtesan

        and then **two strangers** in a hotel bar

            and then . . .
                    In the envelope I left you my suggestion.

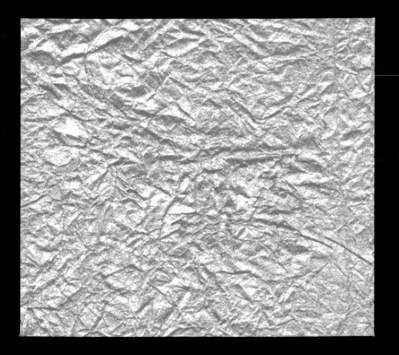

Dissolve your whole body into vision,
so to become seeing, seeing, seeing . . .

Rumi
(thirteenth century)

*I*n the mysterious **darkness**
　　　　my mind can't untangle the clues
　　　　　its search for certainty
　　　　　　　led astray by my imagination

　　　my eyes are **silent**
　　　　　the sum of my sensations focus

　　　　I hear **ecstasy** all around my body

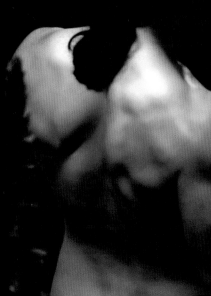

Stand in the middle of the room, with your legs spread.
Then put your hands together, over your head, palm to palm,
with a dime between each pair of fingers and your thumbs.

Pulse beating fast, I thought, what interesting
little game does he have in mind this time? . . .

I walked across the bare wooden boards where he had rolled up the fluffy
rug and stood, legs spread, nipples tightening with excitement as I wondered
what he had planned. I carefully balanced a dime on the tip of each finger
and the thumb of my left hand. Then I put my right hand over the left,
fingertip to fingertip, and raised my arms over my head. He took his
time walking over to me, although his erection advertised that he was
excited, too. He put one hand on my waist and began to walk around
me slowly as he explained,

No matter what I do, no matter how
you feel, don't let go of the dimes.

He was behind me now, his left
arm wrapped around my waist
and his right hand lifting the
long hair from my neck. He
whispered in my ear:

If you drop a dime, and you
can be sure I'll hear it on
this wooden floor,
everything stops . . .
everything.

Anita Mashman

"Five Dimes"

I want to play a game with you . . .

I await your instructions.

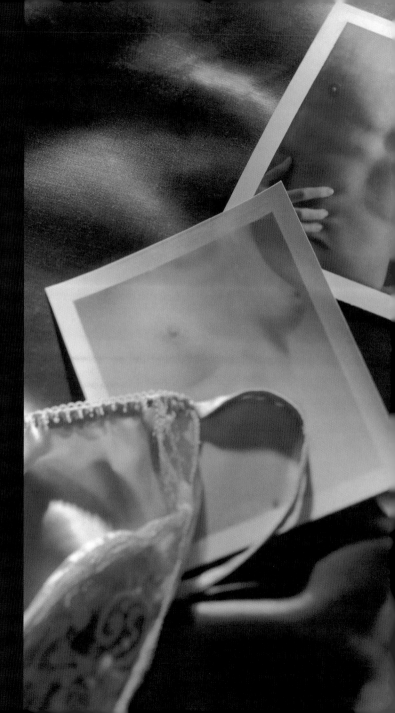

offering us for a minute
the glimpse of
an eternity that we should
like to stretch out
over the whole of time

Albert Camus

POLARO

I've left the camera next to the bed

capture us on film

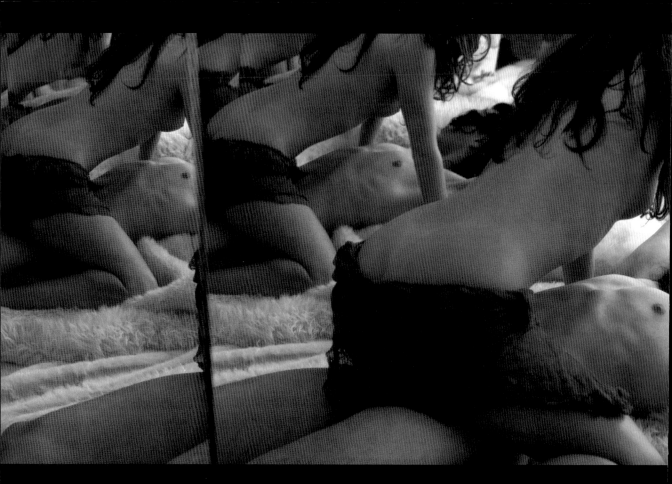

We look at each other in the mirror. She's fascinated. I pull the wrap up over her ass so that she can have a better look. I lift her up and she twines her legs around me. "Yes, do it," she begs. "Fuck me! Fuck me!" Suddenly she untwines her legs, unhitches. She grabs the big armchair and turns it around, resting her hands on the back of it. Her ass is stuck out invitingly. She doesn't wait for me to put it in—she grabs it and places it herself, watching all the time through the mirror.

Henry Miller

Sexus

My eyes follow your every curve

looking straight at you

while **devouring** you from behind

*Sex must be
mixed with
tears,
laughter,
words,
promises,
scenes,
jealousy,
envy,
all the spices
of fear,
foreign travel,
new faces,
novels,
stories,
dreams,
fantasies . . .*

Anaïs Nin
Delta of Venus

*E*ighteenth-century French courtesans, known for their sexual ingenuity and experimentation, were offered a life in the opera if they gave up selling their sexual favors. Let's imagine we found the personal trunk of one of these opera starlets. What secrets would it contain?

Look in the envelope . . .

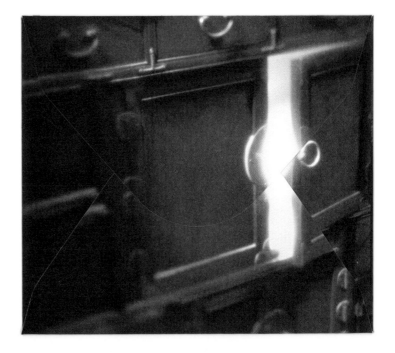

Passing the closet, I couldn't help but notice
three colored boxes stacked on the floor, so I
switched on the light and went in. On top of the
boxes was a note written in big letters: OPEN THE
BOXES AND WEAR ONE OF THE THINGS INSIDE.
I was definitely snared; my curiosity was piqued.

I rummaged through them, and, all in all,
I must admit that he showed some imagination.
In the first box was lingerie, pure white and lacy:
a sheer slip, panties that were at once sensual and
chaste, a push-up bra. Another note placed
inside said, FOR A BABY WHO NEEDS TO BE
CUDDLED. First box rejected.

The second box contained a pink G-string
with some feathers attached behind it, quite like
a rabbit's tail, a pair of fishnet stockings, pink
shoes with vertiginous high heels, and another
note: FOR A BUNNY WHO WANTS TO BE
CAPTURED BY THE HUNTER. Before I rejected it,
I wanted to see what the third box would yield.

I liked this game, this unveiling of his desires.

The third box is what I chose: a shiny black
bodysuit in latex, accompanied by long high-
heeled leather boots, a whip, a black dildo, and
a tube of Vaseline. Apart from the cosmetics, the
box also contained a note that read: FOR A
MISTRESS WHO WANTS TO PUNISH HER SLAVE.
There could be no punishment better than this;
he himself had proposed the means.

Melissa P.
100 Strokes of the Brush Before Bed

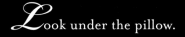ook under the pillow.

I've left you **three envelopes.**
Three different sexual scenarios that we could share.
Each revealing in its own way.

Don't open them yet.
Take your time—read them slowly.

Now pick one.

Which of my three wishes will you choose?

When I closed my own eyes I could imagine
it was her hand upon me, and I did.
"That's so beautiful," she whispered.
"Thank you for letting me watch."
"I've never done this before,"
I managed to mutter.
"Done what?"
I didn't know what to call it.
"This." "What?"
"I've never masturbated,"
I said.
"Neither have I." . . .
"Open your eyes," she said.
"Look at me."
I looked into her eyes
looking at my hand
and tried even to see
the reflection of
myself in them.

J. D. Landis
Lying in Bed

Our wondering eyes are upon each other
rhythm and touch begin
each movement announcing the next
pushing closer—my body tightening
heightening **the anticipation**
knowing **you're next**

Watch me . . . then I'll watch you

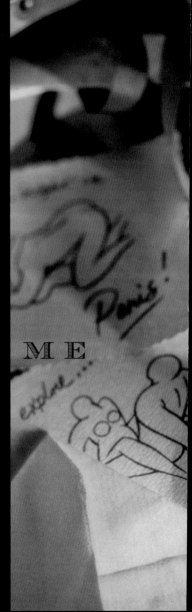

SURPRISE ME

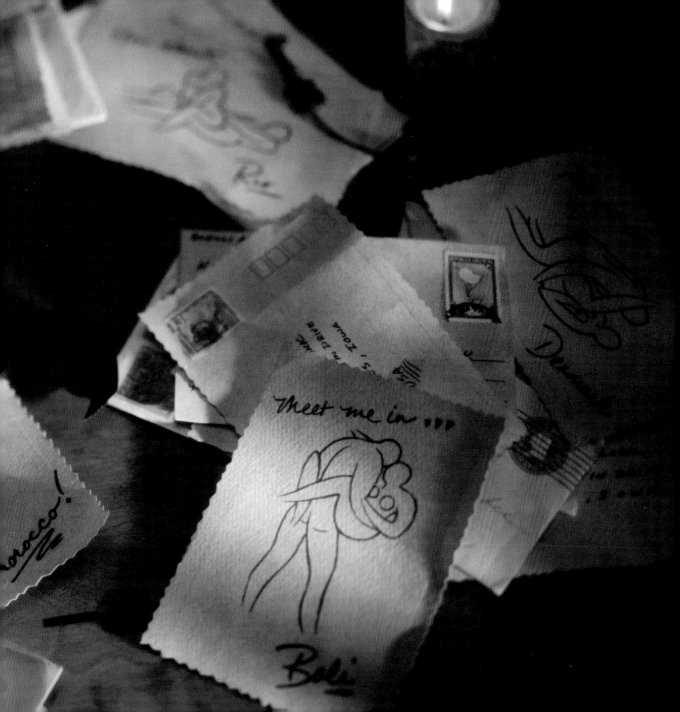

Sex is a key to doorways of knowing.
For me it has been a yoga through
which new qualities of self evolved.
Like the alchemist who works with
potions for decades and in the process
brings about a transmutation of his
essence, I have spent all my conscious
life . . . mixing elements in the crucible
of sex, sifting enormous amounts of
material to produce a few grams of
pure substance. After completing
the entire route, I find it was all
simply a doorway to devotion.

Marco Vassi

*F*or thousands of years, the winds of time have passed over this earth, whispering the sacred knowledge of love. They speak of *maithuna*—the centuries-old Sanskrit word for the highest spiritual and sexual union. Let us continue our quest by exploring the sexual secrets and techniques of the world's different cultures, and see where it may take us.

She felt the soft bud of him within her stirring, and strange rhythms flushing up into her with a strange rhythmic growing motion, swelling and swelling till it filled all her cleaving consciousness, and then began again the unspeakable motion that was not really motion, but pure deepening whirlpools of sensation swirling deeper and deeper through all of her tissue and consciousness, till she was one perfect concentric fluid of feeling.

D. H. Lawrence
Lady Chatterly's Lover

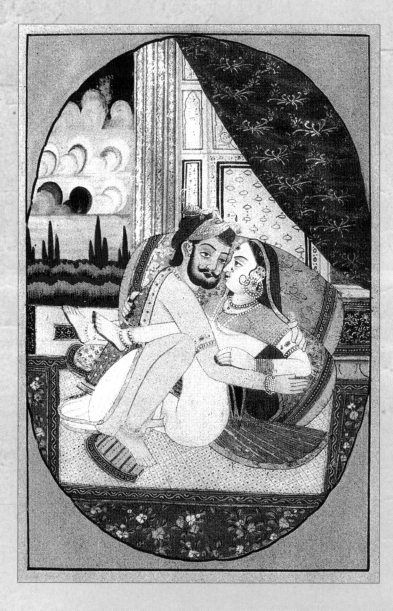

Mixing elixirs
    Yin and Yang—
    a rhythmic combination
    where the man enters the woman and teases her with
    NINE short strokes and then
    ONE deep.

    One then nine.

    One then nine.

"Get in," he says . . .

The taxi moves off slowly, the man still not having said a word to the driver. But he pulls down the shades of the windows on both sides of the car, and the shade on the back window. She has taken off her gloves, thinking he wants to kiss her or that he wants her to caress him. But instead he says:

"Your bag's in your way; let me have it."

She gives it to him. He puts it out of her reach and adds:

"You also have on too many clothes. Unfasten your stockings and roll them down to above your knees. Here are some garters."

By now the taxi has picked up speed, and she has some trouble managing it; she's also afraid the driver may turn around. Finally, though, the stockings are rolled down, and she's embarrassed to feel her legs naked and free beneath her silk slip. Besides, the loose garter-belt suspenders are slipping back and forth.

"Unfasten your garter belt," he says, "and take off your panties."

Pauline Réage
Story of O

*L*ike the candle controls the flame, I am caught in
   your gaze.

Your eyes **take charge**
and I feel a certain calm as you
                    make up the rules.

Are you comfortable?
        Sure . . . I would tell you.
How would I know?
        I'll use the word **red**.

Okay. If you say **red**,
        I'll stop.
But if you say "stop"—
        I'll keep going.

Obscene words have a great capacity for summoning emotions. They awaken passion. If the human being does not use them, he prevents himself from experiencing vividly and truly his sexual nature. He hampers the harmonious evolution of his erotic life. He frustrates the spontaneous integration of all the manifestations of instinct in the supreme blossoming of orgasm.

To reach ecstasy in a natural fashion, it is necessary, then, to break the silence.

Ariel C. Arango
Dirty Words

The erotic soul is both light and dark, two halves entwined, one often

overshadowing the other.

I imagine **your words**, given voice **in the night**,
your erotic **dreams**, the darker language of love.

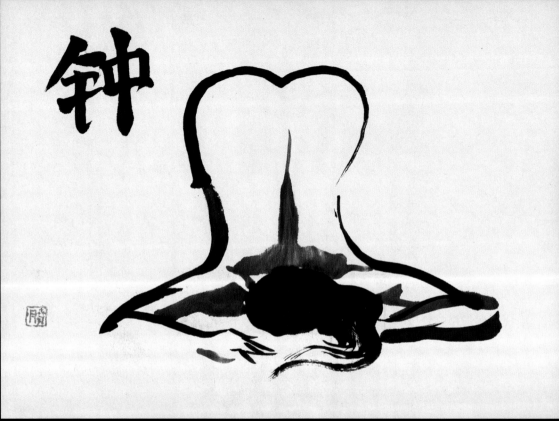

I return to her, running my hands over her lush, wonderfully overflowing cheeks.
"You have such a beautiful ass, I'm surprised it's not permanently red from being
spanked all the time. How can one resist?" I lean close to her and whisper,
biting her neck as I do, feeling the shiver travel down her back.

Rachel Kramer Bussel
"X2"

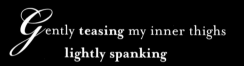

*G*ently **teasing** my inner thighs

    lightly spanking

        for what seems like an eternity . . .

And then that **slap**—

so painful that I could have an orgasm

                every time

*With his head resting between her thighs,
the Adept drinks deeply from the source of
life. Above, the goddess causes his power to
grow and transform into Buddha-fields
within her mind. Below, the Adept endows
each Wave of Wisdom with his means. Each
meditating on the transcendental experience
of non-duality, the confluence of rivers
swells and bursts its banks; there are no
limitations anymore.*

Chandamaharosana Tantra

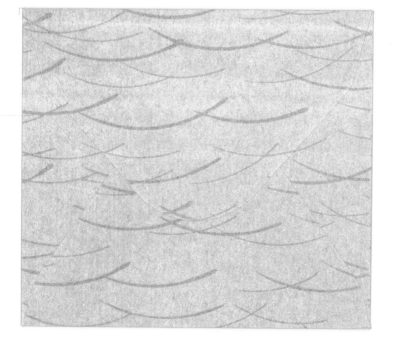

*I*magine feeling
    the softness of **your lips**
pure sensuality
    and **intense pleasure**
your strange **rhythmic motions**
    swirling deeper and deeper
leading me to **explosive sexuality . . .**

Look in the envelope

I see myself, tied to the bed, tied to the dining room table, tied to the legs of the bathroom sink, flushed amid the steam while he takes a shower; I listen to the water roar, sweat beads itching on my upper lip, my eyes closed, my mouth open; tied and stripped, tied and reduced to a single frenzy: craving more.

Elizabeth McNeill
Nine and a Half Weeks

TIE ME UP

I wonder about sensations
   that lie beyond our experience
   imagining how it might feel
   if you quickly tied my wrists

                indulge my curiosity

Then the quivering became a quake,

An eruption, the layers dividing and subdividing.

The quaking broke open into an ancient horizon

Of light and silence,

which opened onto a plane of music and colors

and innocence and longing,

and I felt connection calling connection . . .

Eve Ensler
The Vagina Monologues

The fulfillment of **the ultimate union**

filling all consciousness

as we lie **overcome together**

I'll hold back

until **you're** right there **with me**

If you really make love, all civilization will have to be
dropped. Your mind will have to be put aside—your religion,
philosophy, everything. Suddenly, you will feel like a wild
animal is born within you. A roar will come to you. You
may start actually roaring like a wild animal—screaming,
groaning. And if you allow it, language will disappear.
Sounds will be there, just like birds or animals making
sounds. Suddenly, the whole civilization of a million
years is dropped. You are again standing like an
animal, in a wild world.

Osho
My Way: The Way of the White Clouds

*M*ake love to me

Life leads the thoughtful person on a path of many windings. Now the course is checked, now it runs straight again. Here winged thoughts may pour freely forth in words. There the heavenly burden of knowledge must be shut away in silence. But when two people are as one in their innermost hearts, they shatter even the strength of iron and bronze. And when two people understand each other in their innermost thoughts, their words are sweet and strong, like the fragrance of orchids.

I Ching
hexagram 13, changing line 5

PRIVATE COLLECTION

*L*overs in ancient China often kept pillow books of erotica to honor and inspire their relationships.

They kept them by the bed in wooden boxes decorated with brocade, jade, and silk,

and they took turns filling the pages with words and images of sexual love:

passages from erotic novels, love poems,

quotations from various texts, and drawings of nude scenes and unusual sexual positions.

I've placed a journal next to the bed.

Read my first entry, then add yours to the pages of our private collection.

Let us follow our imagination to live in dreams awake.

Therein lies the promise of a journey that will never end.

"Private Collection" is the fortieth fantasy in the book and the last of this journey.

Throughout history, journeys involving the number 40 have been considered sacred.

THE AUTHORS

WRITE ME A LOVE LETTER
Sei Shonagon, *The Pillow Book of Sei Shonagon* (excerpt), translated and edited by Ivan Morris, Columbia University Press, 1991.

SLOW DANCE
M.L.E. Moreau de Saint-Méry, "Dance," *Repertory of Colonial Information*, 1796. Published by Dance Horizons, 1975. Reprinted by permission of Princeton Book Company.

READ TO ME
Dante Alighieri, *Inferno*, Canto V, translated by Dante Gabriel Rossetti, 1862.

ONE ROMANTIC EVENING
Ananga Ranga, translated by Sir Richard F. Burton, 1885.

SNUGGLE
William S. Burroughs, *Queer*, Penguin Books, 1985.

Pablo Neruda, "Sonnet XVII," in *Into the Garden: A Wedding Anthology*, translated by Stephen Mitchell, copyright © 1993. Published by HarperCollins.

ONLINE INVITATION
Great Dialogues of Plato (Signet Classics), © 1956 by John Cline Graves Rouse. Published by New American Library, a division of Penguin Putnam, Inc.

MASSAGE
Sheik Nefzawi, *The Perfumed Garden*, translated by Sir Richard Burton, 1886.

A CANDLELIT BATH
© Brenda S. Peterson, "Sex As Compassion," in *Nature and Other Mothers*, Ballantine Books, 1995. Reprinted by permission of the author.

SURPRISE ME
Pyotr Ilyich Tchaikovsky, "To My Best Friend": *Correspondence between Tchaikovsky and Nadezhda von Meck,*

1876–1878, edited by Edward Garden and Nigel Gotteri, Clarendon Press, 1993. Reprinted by permission of Oxford University Press.

BREAKFAST IN BED
Maya Angelou, "Where We Belong, A Duet," from *Complete Collected Poems of Maya Angelou*, Random House, 1994.

KISS ME ALL OVER
Alina Reyes, *The Butcher*, Vintage, 1988. Reprinted by permission of The Random House Group Ltd.

LOOK SEXY
Jules Barbey D'Aurevilly in *Feu d'Amour: Seductive Smoke* by Michael Koetzle, © 1994, Benedikt Taschen Verlag GmbH. Reprinted by permission of Benedikt Taschen Verlag GmbH.

Bernard Rudofsky, *The Unfashionable Human Body*, Doubleday, 1971.

LOVEMAKING WITH OIL
The Love Teachings of Kama Sutra, translated by Indra Sinha, Marlowe and Company, 1997.

PHONE SEX
Nicholson Baker, *Vox*, Random House, 1993.

LOVE POTION
Ovid, *The Art of Love (Ars Amatoria)*, translated by A. S. Kline, self-published electronic edition, 2001, www.adkline.freeuk.com/Artoflovehome.htm.

Tung Hsuan Tzu, in *Art of the Bedchamber: The Chinese Sexual Yoga Classics Including Women's Solo Meditation Texts* by Douglas Wile, State University of New York Press, 1992.

THE LOVERS' DANCE
Daniel Odier, *Tantric Quest: An Encounter with Absolute Love*, 1996.

Published by Inner Traditions International, 1997. Reprinted by permission of The Joy Harris Literary Agency, Inc., and Inner Traditions International.

EROTIC MOVIE
Bernardo Bertolucci, *Last Tango in Paris*, screenplay, 1973.

STRIPTEASE
Gustave Flaubert, *The Temptation of Saint Anthony*, translated by Lafcadio Hearn, Modern Library, 2002.

MARSHMALLOW LOVE TUB
Anthony Bourdain, *A Cook's Tour: In Search of the Perfect Meal*, Bloomsbury, 2001. Reprinted by permission of Bloomsbury Publishing.

POSITIONS
Chang Heng Ch'i-pieu, *The Ch'uan-shang-ku-san-ch'in-han-san-kuo-liu-ch'ao-wen Prose Anthology*, compiled by Yen K'o-chun (1762–1843). Privately printed. Translated by Zhenhu Han (1999) and used under license.

ANOTHER WORLD
Anonymous, yen-shih poem, in Valentin Chu, *The Yin-Yang Butterfly: Ancient Chinese Sexual Secrets for Western Lovers*, Putnam, 1993. Reprinted by permission of Valentin Chu.

Marguerite Duras, *The Lover*, Random House, 1985. Reprinted by permission of Random House Inc.

DINNER IS SERVED
Giacomo Casanova di Seingalt, *The Complete Memoirs of Jacques Casanova de Seingalt 1725–1798*. The unabridged London limited edition, translated by Arthur Machen. Privately printed, 1894.

LET'S PRETEND
Virginia Woolf, excerpt from *Orlando*, copyright © 1928 by Virginia Woolf and renewed 1956 by Leonard Woolf.

E. M. Forster, *A Room with a View*, 1908.

BLINDFOLD ME
Rumi in *Sexual Secrets: The Alchemy of Ecstasy* by Nik Douglas and Penny Slinger, Destiny Books, 1979. Reprinted by permission of Inner Traditions International.

GAMES
Anita Mashman, "Five Dimes," in *The Best American Erotica 1993*, Macmillan, 1993. © 1992 by Anita Mashman. Reprinted by permission of author.

POLAROIDS
Albert Camus, *Notebooks 1935–1951*, Marlowe and Company, 1998.

MIRRORS
Henry Miller, *Sexus*, 1965. Used by permission of Grove/Atlantic, Inc. © 1965 by Grove Press, Inc.

SEXUAL TOYS
Anaïs Nin, *Delta of Venus*, Reprinted by permission of Author's Representative Barbara W. Stuhlmann. All rights reserved. Copyright © 1969 by Anaïs Nin. Copyright © 1977 by The Anaïs Nin Trust.

THREE WISHES
Melissa P., *100 Strokes of the Brush Before Bed*, Grove Press, 2004. English translation copyright © 2004 by Lawrence Venuti; copyright © 2003 by Fazi Editore. Reprinted by permission of Thomas Fazi/Fazi Editore.

WATCH ME
J. D. Landis, *Lying in Bed*,

Algonquin Books. Copyright © 1995 by J. D. Landis.

QUEST

Marco Vassi, *The Erotic Impulse: Honoring the Sensual Self*, 1992. Reprinted courtesy of The Permanent Press, Sag Harbor, New York.

Bob Marley, *Bob Marley: In His Own Words*, Omnibus Press, 1993.

ONE THEN NINE

D. H. Lawrence, *Lady Chatterly's Lover*, 1928.

TAKE CONTROL

Pauline Réage, *Story of O*, copyright © 1965 by Grove Press, Inc.

TALK DIRTY TO ME

Ariel C. Arango, *Dirty Words: The Expressive Power of Taboo*, pp. 149–50. Copyright © by Jason Aronson Inc., 1989. Reprinted by permission of Jason Aronson, Inc., and the author. Originally published as *Dirty Words: Psychoanalytic Insights*.

SPANKING

Rachel Kramer Bussel. Originally published in the story "X2" in *Naughty Spanking Stories from A to Z*. Copyright © 2004 by Rachel Kramer Bussel. Published by Pretty Things Press. Reprinted by permission of author.

GOING DOWN

Candramahârosana Tantra, edited and translated by Christopher S. George, American Oriental Society, University of Michigan, 1974.

Hsi Lai, *The Sexual Teachings of the White Tigress: Secrets of the Female Taoists Masters*. Copyright © 2001 by Hsi Lai. Published by Destiny Books. Reprinted by permission of Inner Traditions International.

TIE ME UP

Elizabeth McNeill, *Nine and a Half Weeks*. Reprinted by permission of The Wendy Weil Agency, Inc. First published by E. P. Dutton. Copyright © 1978 by Elizabeth McNeill.

COME TOGETHER

Eve Ensler, "The Vagina Workshop," *The Vagina Monologues*, Villard Books, 1998. Reprinted by permission of Villard Publishers and the author.

MAKE LOVE TO ME

Osho, *My Way: The Way of the White Clouds*. Copyright © 1975 by Osho International Foundation, Switzerland. All rights reserved. Reprinted by arrangement with Osho International Foundation. www.osho.com

PRIVATE COLLECTION

I Ching, hexagram 13, changing line 5. Translated by Richard Wilhelm and Cary F. Baynes, Princeton University Press, 1967. Reprinted by permission of publisher.

ACKNOWLEDGMENTS

This book would not exist without the extraordinary efforts of so many people.

We are indebted to Rinat Aldema, Michael Carlisle, Michele Clement, Frank Curtis, Nik Douglas, Susan Ellinger, Nancy Galdo, Barrie Gillies, Debra Goldstein, Frances Jones, Linda Marso, Grace Moon, Pamela Painter, Silvia Royer, Lisa Shotland, Jonathan Trumper, Norma Wilson, and Eric Zohn.

We also wish to thank the following people for their valuable contributions and support—James Adams, Jerry Basserman, Tony and Sarah Berman, Kandy Bowen, Michael Carabetta, An-Ting Chung, Krystina Clarke, Mary Coleman, Linda Cox, Catherine Cuzzone, Jose Davila, Laura Dean, Tony Edelstein, Erin, Richard Fermeglia, The Firth family, Richard Gerics, Debbie L. Goldman, Donna Goldman, Cheryl Green, Andy Gryn, Sarah Hall, Allyson Hayes, Jennifer Hollier, Lori Jones, Betty Kelly, Karen Kuhen, René Lavallèe, Sally Lewis, Andrea Martin, Daniel Muller, Yoko Nakagawa, Karen O'Shea, Jean Pagliuso, Kate Painter, Melissa Pipe, George Pitts, Allison Prouty, Rebecca Sheehan, John and Brenda Shelly, Swami T., Patti Tateo, Deena Rae Turner, Ed Victor, Maria W. Wade, Sandy Weston, and Roberta Whiting.

We would like to thank all those at Clarkson Potter who gave so much to this project, especially Bill Adams, Doris Cooper, Aliza Fogelson, Maria Gagliano, Adrienne Jozwick, Pam Krauss, Christopher Pavone, Marysarah Quinn, Adina Steiman, and Campbell Wharton.

I would like to thank Susan Ellinger for your creativity and the tireless hours that you gave to this project, Catherine for your wisdom and support, Larry for your friendship and guidance, Mom and Dad for teaching me that anything is possible, and to finish what I started, and Sian for your love and inspiration and for reawakening this project.
—DR

Thank you to my family and friends for your love and support. With regards to this book, I must thank the following individuals for their tremendous contribution—Darcy Raymond, Clay Scheff, Steve "Iceman" Borne, Lukasz "Dr. Luke" Gottwald, Linda Marso, John Wehrheim, Phil and Ashley Jones, Eric Landau, Esther Malamud, Glenn Silver, and Norma Wilson.
—GS